Cambridge Elements ≡

Elements in Emergency Neurosurgery
edited by
Nihal Gurusinghe
Lancashire Teaching Hospital NHS Trust
Peter Hutchinson
University of Cambridge, Society of British Neurological Surgeons and Royal College of Surgeons of England
Ioannis Fouyas
Royal College of Surgeons of Edinburgh
Naomi Slator
North Bristol NHS Trust
Ian Kamaly-Asl
Royal Manchester Children's Hospital
Peter Whitfield
University Hospitals Plymouth NHS Trust

THE CHALLENGES
OF ON-CALL
NEUROSURGERY

Abteen Mostofi
St George's University Hospital

Marco Lee
Stanford University

Nihal Gurusinghe
Lancashire Teaching Hospital NHS Trust

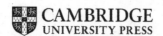

CAMBRIDGE
UNIVERSITY PRESS

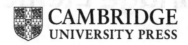

Shaftesbury Road, Cambridge CB2 8EA, United Kingdom

One Liberty Plaza, 20th Floor, New York, NY 10006, USA

477 Williamstown Road, Port Melbourne, VIC 3207, Australia

314–321, 3rd Floor, Plot 3, Splendor Forum, Jasola District Centre, New Delhi – 110025, India

103 Penang Road, #05–06/07, Visioncrest Commercial, Singapore 238467

Cambridge University Press is part of Cambridge University Press & Assessment, a department of the University of Cambridge.

We share the University's mission to contribute to society through the pursuit of education, learning and research at the highest international levels of excellence.

www.cambridge.org
Information on this title: www.cambridge.org/9781009454308

DOI: 10.1017/9781009384520

First published 2023

A catalogue record for this publication is available from the British Library

ISBN 978-1-009-45430-8 Hardback
ISBN 978-1-009-38451-3 Paperback
ISSN 2755-0656 (online)
ISSN 2755-0648 (print)

Cambridge University Press & Assessment has no responsibility for the persistence or accuracy of URLs for external or third-party internet websites referred to in this publication and does not guarantee that any content on such websites is, or will remain, accurate or appropriate.

Every effort has been made in preparing this Element to provide accurate and up-to-date information which is in accord with accepted standards and practice at the time of publication. Although case histories are drawn from actual cases, every effort has been made to disguise the identities of the individuals involved. Nevertheless, the authors, editors and publishers can make no warranties that the information contained herein is totally free from error, not least because clinical standards are constantly changing through research and regulation. The authors, editors and publishers therefore disclaim all liability for direct or consequential damages resulting from the use of material contained in this Element. Readers are strongly advised to pay careful attention to information provided by the manufacturer of any drugs or equipment that they plan to use.

The Challenges of On-Call Neurosurgery

Elements in Emergency Neurosurgery

DOI: 10.1017/9781009384520
First published online: October 2023

Abteen Mostofi
St George's University Hospital

Marco Lee
Stanford University

Nihal Gurusinghe
Lancashire Teaching Hospital NHS Trust

Author for correspondence: Nihal Gurusinghe, nihalgurusinghe@aol.com

Abstract: On-call neurosurgery concerns practice related to urgent and emergency neurosurgical care including outside of 'normal' working hours. Being on call involves many competing responsibilities and is regarded as one of the most demanding aspects of a neurosurgical career. The on-call work pattern has evolved over the past decade due to changes in demographics, technology and working practices, each of which have brought new and emerging challenges. These challenges aside, the on call provides a unique and rewarding environment to make a meaningful difference to patients and to learn the science and art of neurosurgery. Success in on-call work requires not only good technical knowledge and application but also a wide variety of non-technical skills. These skills will help in dealing with some of the difficult situations neurosurgeons in training face when on call, making the experience more manageable and educational.

Keywords: challenges, emergency, neurosurgery, on call, preparation

ISBNs: 9781009454308 (HB), 9781009384513 (PB), 9781009384520 (OC)
ISSNs: 2755-0656 (online), 2755-0648 (print)

Contents

It's 9 a.m. on a Saturday morning and I'm on call for neurosurgery (Figure 1).

The junior in the team is a locum who started yesterday and has no experience in neurosurgery!

Already there have been three referral calls with urgent problems. A patient with cauda equina syndrome admitted early this morning is due to undergo an emergency operation. I am eager to do the operation but because of my limited experience the on-call consultant has kindly agreed to come in and assist me.

A patient who had a craniotomy yesterday is unwell on the ward. I really need to fit in a ward round to assess her and, in addition, to ensure all is well with the other patients.

I also need to speak to a relative who is upset because his mother's operation for a chronic subdural haematoma was cancelled yesterday because of another emergency.

I need to find a source on spontaneous intracerebral haemorrhage for the tutorial I am presenting on Monday if time allows, which right now seems unlikely.

And I had no time to prepare my usual packed lunch today!

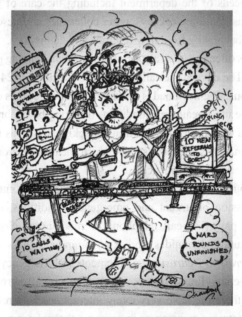

Figure 1 On-call trainee at work not adequately prepared for the challenges (with kind permission of Dr Chandru Kaliaperumal).

1 Introduction to On-Call Neurosurgery

It is estimated that 50 per cent or more of the caseload in neurosurgery relates to emergency and urgent conditions [1]. The mechanism by which most departments cater for this is the 'on-call service'. What constitutes the on-call service naturally varies by country, health-care system and individual department. In most settings, it involves a dedicated clinician or team of clinicians in training ('registrars' or 'residents', depending on the system), under the supervision of a qualified specialist ('consultant' or 'attending' neurosurgeon), specifically delegated the responsibility of dealing with emergency and urgent work. Within such a team, members may take on different roles. For example, a junior trainee (Postgraduate Year (PGY) 1/2 in the USA or Specialist Trainee (ST) 1/2 in the UK) may primarily manage ward-based care of inpatients, while one or more senior trainees (PGY3+ or ST3+) take responsibility for new referrals, emergency admissions and emergency operations. In reality, the 'team' also includes a wider group of clinical and other professionals such as anaesthetists, intensivists, radiologists, theatre nurses and so on.

How the on-call service functions, even within a department, can differ depending on the day of the week and time of day. For example, the on-call team may face additional responsibilities outside of 'normal working hours' (i.e., during evenings, nights and weekends) as they are the only available clinicians for all the medical needs of the department including the care of ward or 'floor' patients. In contrast, during weekdays, other colleagues are present to deal with work other than that arising from new referrals and admissions.

Being on call is often regarded as one of the most challenging parts of training in neurosurgery. The days are usually long (12 or sometimes 24 hours) and the pressure continuous. The workload is considerable, and the cases encountered are varied and include life-threatening conditions requiring both a broad knowledge of the specialty as well as an ability to triage quickly the serious from the trivial. Stress is compounded by the high stakes which mean that wrong decisions or delays can have serious consequences.

Much of the burden of the on call is in being the first point of contact for referral or discussion of urgent and emergency conditions, usually via the dreaded 'bleep', pager, on-call telephone or more novel electronic referral systems (see Grundy, Joannides and Ray, *Sources, Modes and Triage of Emergency Referrals to Neurosurgery*, Elements in Emergency Neurosurgery, Cambridge University Press, forthcoming). The on-call surgeon in a busy department may therefore have very many interactions with referring teams – via telephone, electronic message or in person – throughout a working day. In the authors' departments this typically amounts to as many as 100 interactions in a 24-hour period. This continuous state of being 'in-demand' is the source of much human frustration for referring colleagues who can spend a great deal of time trying to make contact during busy periods – frustration which can be directed back at the on-call neurosurgeon.

Despite the challenges, the on call is uniquely educational, and the rewards can be huge – for example, in the many cases where timely action and intervention is life-saving. The job involves many competing responsibilities, an important selection of which are summarised in Box 1.

BOX 1 RESPONSIBILITIES OF THE ON-CALL TRAINEE/TEAM

Clinical

- Referrals (internally, and from a network of referring hospitals)
- Admissions
- Ward rounds
- Unwell or deteriorating inpatients
- Emergency operations
- Contemporaneous documentation

Administration

- Bed prioritisation/patient flow
- Booking urgent operations on theatre lists

Team-related

- Training of junior colleagues
- Supporting junior/nursing/critical care colleagues
- Discussion with senior colleagues

Personal

- Nutrition and hydration
- Attending to bodily functions
- Dealing with stressful or upsetting situations
- Maintaining own physical and mental health

Communication

- With consultant (now versus at a convenient time)
- With referring teams
- With colleagues
- With patients and relatives (including breaking bad news)
- Consenting for procedures
- Updating handover documentation

The challenge of on-call neurosurgery is to juggle these demands in such a way as to maximise the quality of care delivered to patients within the constraints of limited time and resources. Yet the job is also unmistakably human, and so compassion towards patients and relatives, as well as respect for colleagues in often stressful and difficult circumstances, is paramount. In addition to all the essential technical neurosurgical knowledge, to succeed requires a delicate synthesis of planning and prioritisation of duties based on clinical urgency, strategies that facilitate efficient working without compromising quality or safety and effective communication skills.

In this Element we explore how on-call neurosurgery has been changing over the years, the new specific challenges that this has brought to the job and discuss some strategies that could foster efficiency and help deal with some of the difficulties. The examples used reflect mainly the authors' experience of the UK National Health Service (NHS) and the USA but may apply equally to other systems.

2 The Changing Shape of On-Call Neurosurgery

On-call neurosurgery has undergone a significant transformation over recent decades. One of the ongoing challenges is that the overall number of new urgent and emergency referrals has increased and continues to do so. We speculate on a number of potential factors that have contributed to this and these are discussed in this section. Furthermore, in some health-care systems, working conditions have been significantly reformed, leading to major changes in the way on-call services are structured.

2.1 Trauma Care and Changing Demographics

The demographics of trauma have changed markedly over the past few decades. Historically, trauma was a problem predominantly affecting young men in high-energy incidents such as road traffic collisions; however, the ageing population and improved road safety mean that it is now predominated by low-energy falls in an increasingly elderly and comorbid cohort in whom acute neurosurgical intervention is often not indicated [2]. Also, the increasing use of e-scooters and quad bikes has resulted in another mode of severe injury on the roads involving both riders and pedestrians.

The introduction of major trauma centres, universality of computed tomography (CT) in the emergency setting and strict imaging guidelines have all resulted in increased scanning and detection of brain and spine pathology that may previously have gone undetected. Although the incidence of traumatic injuries requiring emergency neurosurgical intervention is declining [3], this does not seem to have diminished the on-call neurosurgeon's role, as the volume of urgent referrals to neurosurgery is increasing [4, 5]. While in the vast majority of cases these acute injuries do not warrant immediate admission or specialist management in a neurosurgical centre, increasing low-energy trauma in the elderly may well be a substrate for the well-documented increasing burden of surgically managed chronic subdural haematoma [6]. Furthermore, the complex health needs of the increasing elderly population pose unique challenges as coexisting health conditions can complicate overall medical care. For example, the common use of antiplatelet and anticoagulant medication in this group in the context of traumatic intracranial haemorrhage often prompts close liaison between on-call teams and the referring clinicians caring for these patients to manage blood thinning agents based on the perceived balance of risks and benefits (see Poon and Al-Shahi Salman, *Antiplatelet and Anticoagulant Medications and the Emergency Neurosurgical Patient*, Elements in Emergency Neurosurgery, Cambridge University Press, forthcoming).

2.2 Decreased Thresholds for Referral and Advice

In our collective experience, across multiple departments, there has been an apparent lowering of the threshold for referral to and discussion with on-call neurosurgery services over recent decades. In many hospitals, internal medical, general surgical, orthopaedic or trauma teams are required to care for patients who do not or are unlikely to require immediate neurosurgical input. In many centres, particularly in the USA, non-neurosurgical teams can manage these patients very effectively and refer them to neurosurgery when appropriate. However, our perception, particularly in the UK setting, is that: (1) more and more management decisions regarding patients under the care of other non-neurosurgical teams are being deferred to on-call neurosurgery rather than being made locally; and (2) discussions that need not be urgent are being inappropriately expedited outside of normal working hours. These are contributing to the overall rise in workload.

The reasons behind these developments are difficult to elucidate clearly and are likely multifactorial. Potential contributors may include decreased competence or confidence of non-specialist medical teams caring for patients with neurosurgical problems. This is perhaps a result of increasing specialisation in medicine as a whole or it may reflect a deficiency on the part of neurosurgeons in educating and empowering other specialties to manage these patients when urgent neurosurgical intervention is not required (see Section 3.2). A culture of heightened accountability and medicolegal anxiety may be at play, making non-neurosurgical colleagues understandably reluctant to make decisions in respect of problems outside of their specialist remit. This anxiety is perhaps caused by a continued rise in medical litigation and compounded by a small number of recent high-profile cases in which doctors have been criminally convicted for gross negligence. Furthermore, the introduction of electronic referral systems (see Grundy, Joannides and Ray, *Sources, Modes and Triage of Emergency*

Referrals to Neurosurgery, Elements in Emergency Neurosurgery, Cambridge University Press, forthcoming) to replace the traditional method of referral via pager and/or telephone makes referral to and discussion with the on-call neurosurgical team logistically less onerous and more accessible.

We speculate also that increased workloads, particularly in emergency departments, which in the UK have seen an unprecedented rise in attendances in recent years, create a desire for increased specialist support to help assess and manage patients with potential neurosurgical problems. This rise in emergency attendances is partly driven by inappropriate access of emergency departments for non-urgent conditions (for example, degenerative spinal disease), perhaps due to increasingly stretched resources in primary care, diverting what ought to be managed on an elective pathway to the on-call service. Another related factor specific to UK emergency departments may be the application of the 'four-hour target' which mandates that 95 per cent of patients should be admitted, transferred or discharged within four hours of arrival, thereby granting 'logistical urgency' to clinically non-urgent problems.

2.3 Conditions of Employment

The European Working Time Directive (EWTD) comprises a series of minimum requirements in relation to work hours, rest periods and annual leave. Although not necessarily applicable to health-care systems outside of the UK and European Union, its implementation (in 2009 in the UK) has limited the working hours of medical doctors to an average of 48 hours per week, a significant reduction compared to those previously worked by surgeons in training. As individual doctors can now work fewer hours, many departments have responded by increasing resident/registrar numbers in order to provide on-call cover within EWTD-compliant rosters.

These changes in working patterns yield a number of challenges. First, with limits on time at work and the expansion of the resident/registrar grade, there is an impact on training with a risk of reduction in exposure to both elective and emergency neurosurgery. Second, an increase in shift work and clinical handovers between shifts has resulted in the need for effective and robust handover procedures between colleagues on call (see Lammy and Brown, *Duty and Standards of Care: Handovers, Care of Inpatients, Record Keeping and Assessment of Ward Attenders*, Elements in Emergency Neurosurgery, Cambridge University Press, forthcoming). The experience of on-call trainees can be variable and therefore support and supervision from senior colleagues is essential. This is easier to achieve between 9 a.m. and 5 p.m. on weekdays but requires more resources after hours and at weekends.

2.4 Sub-Specialisation

On-call neurosurgery involves both cranial and spinal conditions. On-call teams should have the capability and skill mix to perform emergency operations on a wide range of conditions. Sub-specialisation within neurosurgery has increased over the years and is well established to achieve improved outcomes for elective operations. The same principle probably applies to emergency conditions. The timelines of management for complex spinal surgery have become more stringent and many units have a spinal on-call rota to provide additional support. Similarly, in neuro-vascular surgery, urgent conditions such as a ruptured cerebral aneurysm with a life-threatening haematoma may require sub-specialist surgical support (see Zammit and Nelson, *The Role of Sub-Specialisation in Emergency Neurosurgery*, Elements in Emergency Neurosurgery, Cambridge University Press, forthcoming).

2.5 Different Health-Care Systems

There are additional challenges associated with specific health-care systems. In socialised medicine (e.g., in the UK NHS), on-call activity is driven by the principle of prioritisation based on clinical need (see Lilo and Fouyas, *Clinical Priority for Common Emergency and Urgent Conditions in Neurosurgery*, Elements in Emergency Neurosurgery, Cambridge University Press, forthcoming); however, in market-driven private health-care systems, such as that in the USA, a response to an on-call consultation and its documentation translates into revenue for the service. The promptness of the response may also be 'rewarded' by a higher bill and therefore increased remuneration for the department. This financial incentive puts further pressure on trainees who are obliged by the department to respond to as many consults as possible. In some systems, for example, in parts of North America, there are departments without trainees, and on-call services are provided solely by attending surgeons who face more pressure compared to trainees who may be able to look forward to a less stressful on-call experience after training.

3 Key Strategies to Cope with Challenges

There are a few important skills and tactics that can help with the challenges of the on-call experience. These are summarised in Box 2 and elaborated further in this section.

3.1 Preparation

Before starting an on-call shift, it is important to make certain that you are physically, mentally and logistically prepared. Illness, injury, lack of sleep or

Box 2 Essential survival toolkit

- Workstation with essential equipment
- Preparation and planning
- Working within a team
- Core knowledge
- Communication and interpersonal skills
- Happy work environment
- Personal care

distressing personal circumstances can all have an impact on the ability to perform under stressful conditions on call. It is essential to inform your department at the earliest opportunity and excuse yourself from the shift if you feel unprepared. On the logistical side, ensuring access from the start of the shift to a dedicated and comfortable computer workstation (Figure 2), IT systems, telephone, important telephone and pager numbers, relevant departmental protocols, clinical examination instruments and a ready supply of food and drink will save you much time and increase your efficiency throughout the day.

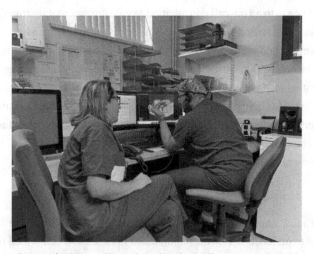

Figure 2 A typical on-call workstation including: a comfortable chair; a computer with appropriate screen size and resolution for viewing images and online referral systems; a telephone and headset; and useful information, guidelines and protocols pinned up on the wall nearby.

3.2 Communication and Interaction with Colleagues

Clinical communication is said to account for the largest share of medical errors [7] and it certainly comprises a huge proportion of the on-call neurosurgeon's work, especially when dealing with a high volume of referrals. Communication with colleagues can be fractious as our priorities as neurosurgeons do not always align with those of referring colleagues, and this can be a source of much friction and dissatisfaction. Examples encountered frequently include disagreements on whether referred patients should be admitted to a neurosurgical centre or managed locally. An increasing number of units now utilise electronic referral systems which act as the medium of communication with referring clinicians and provide a written record of the dialogue that is accessible by both the on-call neurosurgical and referring teams (see Grundy, Joannides and Ray, *Sources, Modes and Triage of Emergency Referrals to Neurosurgery*, Elements in Emergency Neurosurgery, Cambridge University Press, forthcoming).

3.3 Expectation Management

Many frustrations in relation to on-call neurosurgery can be mitigated with effective communication strategies and expectation management, which in the long run will save you time and stress. For example, explanation to referring teams of the reasoning behind decisions, anticipation of future queries and pre-emptive provision of suitable guidance will lead to fewer repeat discussions for the same referral. There will be many situations in which rapid coordinated communication is critical to ensure a good outcome for the patient. For example, arrangement of a typical time-critical emergency transfer to a neurosurgical unit might involve dialogue with multiple individuals including the referring clinician, on-call consultant neurosurgeon, intensivist, anaesthetist, theatre team leader, bed manager, ward charge nurse and, on arrival, the transfer team and patient and/or relatives (see May and Dark, *Admitting a Patient to the Critical Care Unit*, Elements in Emergency Neurosurgery, Cambridge University Press, forthcoming). Ensure that all parties who may need to know about an emergency are informed as early as possible and provided with estimated timings so that they can be available when needed while prioritising and planning their duties accordingly. This avoids both delays in the transfer as well as colleagues' frustration due to feeling that they were unable to prepare for the situation.

Lack of availability to answer calls is a major source of frustration for colleagues. If urgent clinical work, such as being busy performing a surgical procedure or spending time with an unwell patient, means that you will be unable to take referral calls for a prolonged period of time, a number of actions can be taken to mitigate the negative impact on callers. The responsibility could be delegated to another team member such as a junior colleague or theatre nurse. Junior or non-medical colleagues should not be put in a position of giving advice beyond their remit, but at the very least they can explain the situation, ask about the nature and urgency of the call and take contact details so that the caller can be called back at the earliest opportunity. Likewise, the hospital switchboard operator can play an important role in informing external callers of your unavailability if you give them this instruction. Many electronic referral systems also allow information on unavailability to be relayed to referrers. The aim here, again, is expectation management, and it is much better and less frustrating for callers on hold to know that you are busy and for how long you will be unavailable than to wait on the line indefinitely. However, make sure that colleagues who respond to callers are aware of what provisions are in place for those who feel they need help with an emergency situation which really cannot wait until you are available – for example, immediate escalation to the consultant or attending neurosurgeon who should also be pre-emptively informed.

3.4 Dealing with Frustration

On-call neurosurgery is a stressful and often frustrating job, and it is easy to allow this to boil over into unpleasant interactions with referring clinicians and colleagues. Our experience is that, historically, on-call interactions between neurosurgeons and other departments might have been deemed hostile and, indeed, adversarial. Frustration might relate to disagreement with a management plan you have given to a referrer, from an inappropriate referral or having to argue with another specialty (e.g., anaesthetics or radiology) for access to emergency theatres or investigations; this might be compounded by prejudices on both sides arising from perceived 'neurosurgical elitism'. As frustrated as you are, it is essential to maintain professional respect for your colleagues. For example, in the case of a seemingly trivial or inappropriate referral, remember that the majority of colleagues are there to do their best for patients and that there is an unwell patient at the centre of the discussion. If they have contacted you, it is because they feel unable to deal with a clinical problem with which you can potentially help.

Conflict in the workplace is clearly not desirable given the need for effective patient-centred teamwork and we wholeheartedly recommend a move away from an adversarial culture. The art of negotiation is essential here, and to implement this requires calm, objective and persuasive discussion. For example, a referrer unhappy with your suggested management should be given the chance to voice and discuss their specific concerns and be reassured and protected with respect to those concerns, as appropriate. While it may not seem like an efficient use of time during the commotion of the on call, do make use of opportunities to educate referring doctors constructively, without any hint of condescension or disrespect. Education and empowerment will improve the ability of referring specialties to look after patients in the long run, by giving them the know-how to understand when to (and when not to) escalate a problem to on-call neurosurgical services with the appropriate level of urgency. Certainly, outside of the on call, neurosurgical involvement in planned educational activities and the creation of clear guidelines and protocols for referring specialties are strategies that might, in the long-term, reduce the burden of inappropriate referrals to the on-call service.

3.5 Handovers

With the increase in on-call workload and expanding resident/registrar numbers, effective handover communication is becoming more challenging. Most departments have a set process for handover although the levels of formality differ between units. It is essential throughout the shift to keep a meticulous record of important issues to handover, both to the ward teams regarding admissions and unwell patients and to the incoming on-call team for unresolved issues from referrals. In the heat of the moment, it may not seem a priority to update a handover document, but missed handover of an important clinical problem has the potential to result in significant harm to a patient; it should therefore not be taken lightly. The handover often involves patient(s) awaiting an emergency operation and it is important to ensure all relevant clinical details are explained to the new clinical team (see Lammy and Brown, *Duty and Standards of Care: Handovers, Care of Inpatients, Record Keeping and Assessment of Ward Attenders*, Elements in Emergency Neurosurgery, Cambridge University Press, forthcoming).

3.6 Working as a Team and Leadership

The on call is commonly delivered by a team of clinicians. This might include a number of doctors at different stages of training, as well as other frontline health-care professionals such as physician assistants/associates or nurse practitioners. Effective team working and leadership are essential. A senior clinician on the ground should assume the role of team leader to prioritise and delegate responsibilities to each team member in order to maximise efficiency of working. Within the team everyone should be encouraged to express an opinion and feel comfortable about doing so; this is also called 'speaking up for the patient' [8].

The attending or consultant neurosurgeon on call may not be present on site all of the time but carries ultimate responsibility for care delivered by the team. Appropriate discussion with and escalation to the attending/consultant neurosurgeon are essential. Be explicitly aware of their whereabouts and intended movements and the best method for contacting them when needed. To avoid inefficiency, these discussions should be prioritised and held in a timely manner, depending on urgency. Clearly, as knowledge and experience increase through training, so does the ability to prioritise appropriately. Nobody would argue that a discussion regarding a time-critical situation should be delayed. However, less urgent problems which do not require an immediate definitive decision, such as a stable spinal fracture without neurological deficit or a new diagnosis of brain tumour in a stable patient, can be saved for discussion together at a more convenient time later in the day.

3.7 Core Knowledge

Safe decision-making is the fundamental objective when on call and sound basic knowledge of emergency practice is essential (see Moon and Wigfield, *Making Safe Clinical Decisions in Emergency Care*, Elements in Emergency Neurosurgery, Cambridge University Press, forthcoming). In addition to the support offered, a great deal is learnt from the teaching and observing of senior colleagues. One of the advantages of being on call is the unique learning experience. Such knowledge of emergency practice may be extremely helpful in consolidating preparation for examinations. Awareness of common clinical pathways facilitates early and safe decision-making in time-critical situations.

3.8 Personal Care

It is difficult to believe, but even the on-call neurosurgery registrar is human. Prior to starting each shift, it is important to have access to a supply of sustenance. Make sure you take the time to eat and drink, as well as attending to basic bodily functions! Most clinical activities allow you to take some time to do this. As a senior internal physician once said to one of the authors, 'if it can't wait a few minutes, then it doesn't need you, it needs the crash team!'.

You will encounter many tragic and emotive situations in the acute setting. While a degree of desensitisation is both inevitable and arguably necessary in order to have the focus to perform effectively during these situations, it is easy to underestimate the mental health burden and emotional toll that this can take over time. The importance of mental health and well-being is increasingly in the spotlight, especially among frontline health-care workers, and, fortunately, the historical stigma associated with it is fading. Know what sources of support and help are available and be willing to use them. This can be in the form of colleagues with responsibility for pastoral care such as clinical or educational supervisors, formal peer-support or counselling services, the hospital chaplaincy or your own general practitioner. If things do get overwhelming, then be sure to let someone know and take action early before things spiral out of control.

Finally, a congenial and welcoming work environment is a key requirement for effective clinical practice. Unfortunately, bullying and harassment can be a problem in some units and should not be tolerated. Ensure you are aware of local and national policies and the support systems available to raise these issues due to their negative impact on the workplace (see Stovell and Carleton-Bland, *The Work Environment – Human Factors*, Elements in Emergency Neurosurgery, Cambridge University Press, forthcoming).

4 Conclusions

On-call neurosurgery is uniquely challenging yet enormously rewarding, with a vast number of important responsibilities to prioritise in the context of the high stress of an emergency situation. It has undergone many changes due to shifting population demographics and changing working practices and will undoubtedly continue to evolve in response to further developments in the health-care landscape. The workload is increasing and the resulting burden to physical and mental health of working long, tiring and sometimes emotionally charged shifts is high and should not be underestimated. Core knowledge and experience are prerequisites for good clinical decision-making and management. Many perceived difficulties in the role can be reduced with appropriate non-technical skills including preparation, advance planning, teamwork and clear and effective communication with colleagues in a happy working environment.

> *It's 9 a.m. on Saturday morning and I'm on call for neurosurgery (Figure 3).*
>
> *The junior in the team is a locum who started yesterday and fortunately has some experience in neurosurgery.*
>
> *We did an early ward round this morning to resolve some post-op concerns on the ward and made a plan with the charge nurse to speak to a relative who is worried about his mother's condition.*
>
> *I am looking forward to performing the surgery on a patient with cauda equina syndrome at 11 a.m. The consultant will be standing by in case I need help.*
>
> *I have found an online source to prepare for a tutorial on Monday on spontaneous intracerebral haemorrhage.*
>
> *Looking forward to my packed lunch with salad and salmon after the operation . . .*

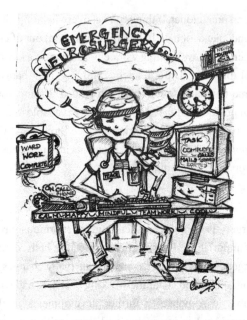

Figure 3 On-call trainee at work calm and prepared for the challenges
(with kind permission from Dr Chandru Kaliaperumal)

References

1. Emergency Surgery: Standards for Unscheduled Surgical Care. The Royal College of Surgeons of England; 2011. https://www.rcseng.ac.uk/library-and-publications/rcs-publications/docs/emergency-surgery-standards-for-unscheduled-care/

2. Kehoe A, Smith JE, Edwards A, Yates D, Lecky F. The changing face of major trauma in the UK. Emerg Med J. 2015;32(12):911–15.

3. Giner J, Mesa Galan L, Yus Teruel S et al. Traumatic brain injury in the new millennium: new population and new management. Neurologia (Engl Ed). 2022;37(5):383–9.

4. Spencer RJ, Amer S, St George EJ. A retrospective analysis of emergency referrals and admissions to a regional neurosurgical centre 2016–2018. Br J Neurosurg. 2021;35(4):438–43.

5. Kennion O, Jayakumar N, Kamal MA et al. Use of an online referral service for acute neurosurgical referrals: an institutional experience. World Neurosurg. 2022; Vol 165, pp. e438–445. DOI: 10.1016/j.wneu.2022.06.071

6. Stubbs DJ, Vivian ME, Davies BM et al. Incidence of chronic subdural haematoma: a single-centre exploration of the effects of an ageing population with a review of the literature. Acta Neurochir (Wien). 2021;163(9):2629–37.

7. Campbell P, Torrens C, Pollock A, Maxwell M. A scoping review of evidence relating to communication failures that lead to patient harm. Nursing, Midwifery and Allied Health Professionals Research Unit; 2018.

8. Syed M. Black Box Thinking (Part 1: A Routine Operation). Penguin Publishing Group; 2015.

Acknowledgement

We are indebted to our colleague for the cartoons (Figures 1 and 3): Dr Chandru Kaliaperumal, DipMedEd, PDCR, FEBNS, FRCSI, FRCSEd(Neuro.Surg), Consultant Paediatric and Adult Neurosurgeon, the Royal Infirmary of Edinburgh & Royal Hospital for Children and Young People, Edinburgh; Honorary Senior Clinical Lecturer, University of Edinburgh Foundation Programme Director, NHS Education for Scotland.

Cambridge Elements ☰

Emergency Neurosurgery

Nihal Gurusinghe
Lancashire Teaching Hospital NHS Trust

Professor Nihal Gurusinghe is a Consultant Neurosurgeon at the Lancashire Teaching Hospitals NHS Trust. He is on the Executive Council of the Society of British Neurological Surgeons as the Lead for NICE (National Institute for Health and Care Excellence) guidelines relating to neurosurgical practice. He is also an examiner for the UK and International FRCS examinations in Neurosurgery.

Peter Hutchinson
University of Cambridge, Society of British Neurological Surgeons and Royal College of Surgeons of England

Peter Hutchinson BSc MBBS FFSEM FRCS(SN) PhD FMedSci is Professor of Neurosurgery and Head of the Division of Academic Neurosurgery at the University of Cambridge, and Honorary Consultant Neurosurgeon at Addenbrooke's Hospital. He is Director of Clinical Research at the Royal College of Surgeons of England and Meetings Secretary of the Society of British Neurological Surgeons.

Ioannis Fouyas
Royal College of Surgeons of Edinburgh

Ioannis Fouyas is a Consultant Neurosurgeon in Edinburgh. His clinical interests focus on the treatment of complex cerebrovascular and skull base pathologies. His academic endeavours concentrate in the field of cerebrovascular pathophysiology. His passion is technical surgical training, fulfilled in collaboration with the Royal College of Surgeons of Edinburgh. Finally, he pursues Undergraduate Neuroscience teaching, with a particular focus on functional Neuroanatomy.

Naomi Slator
North Bristol NHS Trust

Naomi Slator FRCS (SN) is a Consultant Spinal Neurosurgeon based at North Bristol NHS Trust. She has a specialist interest in Complex Spine alongside Cranial and Spinal Trauma. She completed her neurosurgical training in Birmingham and a six-month Fellowship in CSF and Trauma (2019). She then went on to complete her Spinal Fellowship in Leeds (2020) before moving to the southwest to take up her consultant post.

Ian Kamaly-Asl
Royal Manchester Children's Hospital

Ian Kamaly-Asl is a full time paediatric neurosurgeon and Honorary Chair at Royal Manchester Children's Hospital. He trained in North Western Deanery with fellowships at Boston Children's Hospital and Sick Kids in Toronto. Ian is a member of council of The Royal College of Surgeons of England and The SBNS where he is lead for mentoring and tackling oppressive behaviours.

Peter Whitfield

University Hospitals Plymouth NHS Trust

Professor Peter Whitfield is a Consultant Neurosurgeon at the South West Neurosurgical Centre, University Hospitals Plymouth NHS Trust. His clinical interests include vascular neurosurgery, neuro oncology and trauma. He has held many roles in postgraduate neurosurgical education and is President of the Society of British Neurological Surgeons. Peter has published widely, and is passionate about education, training and the promotion of clinical research.

About the Series

Elements in Emergency Neurosurgery is intended for trainees and practitioners in Neurosurgery and Emergency Medicine as well as allied specialties all over the world. Authored by international experts, this series provides core knowledge, common clinical pathways and recommendations on the management of acute conditions of the brain and spine.